Delicious Smoothie Recipes Book For Beginners!

Smoothie Recipes

Feel Great And Get In Shape With 120 Rejuvenating And Essential Smoothies For Detox, Weight Loss And Clean Eating!

Sarah Brooks

Copyright © 2015 Sarah Brooks

STOP!!! Before you read any further....Would you like to know the Secrets of Body Transformation?

If your answer is yes, then you are not alone. Thousands of people are looking for the secret to rapidly burn body fat, keep the weight off, become healthier, and truly transform their body and life for good.

If you have been searching for these answers without much luck, you are in the right place!

Not only will you gain incredible insight in this book, but because I want to make sure to give you as much value as possible, right now for a limited time you can get full **100% FREE access to a VIP bonus EBook** entitled **THE 7 KEYS TO BODY TRANSFORMATION!**

Just Go Here For Free Instant Access:

www.liveFitVIP.com

Legal Notice

Disclaimer Notice

Table Of Contents

Introduction

I want to thank you and congratulate you for purchasing the book, *"Smoothie Recipes: Feel Great And Get In Shape With 120 Rejuvenating And Essential Smoothies For Detox, Weight Loss And Clean Eating!"*

This "Smoothie Recipes" book contains proven steps and strategies on how to make 120 amazingly easy, delicious and healthy smoothies.

In this book, you will learn how to make 120 smoothies at home fit for a king. These include smoothies for weight loss, for radiant skin, for detox, for boosting metabolism and increasing energy, for strengthening the immune system, for alkaline weight loss, and even smoothies for fighting cancers and diseases!

Rest assured, you will not run out of delicious additions to your diet with the help of this recipe book and guide.

Thanks again for purchasing this book, I hope you enjoy it!

Chapter 1 - Smoothies For Beginners

Nowadays, people are so busy that they think they no longer have time to prepare healthy meals at home. Unfortunately, this way of thinking has led them to choose unhealthy options such as fast food. These quick fixes might make one feel fuller for a few hours, but the lack of nutrients in these dishes fail to nourish the body. Eventually, this lifestyle will lead to an unhealthy body that is prone to health issues.

The good news is that there actually is a way to a healthier diet, even if you are in a hurry. One way to give your body the nutrients it needs is by making smoothies. All you will need is a powerful and durable blender.

There are many benefits for choosing to drink up your nutrients.

First, you are getting rid of high-calorie and high-fat foods from your diet.

Second, you are eliminating the "not tasty" factor of certain healthy foods because they will simply slide down your throat.

Third, you are giving your body the fiber it needs because making smoothies still retains the fiber in the ingredients.

Lastly and most importantly, you are nourishing your cells with top-notch nutrients straight from their natural source.

Many nutritionists recommend that you should drink a variety of healthy smoothies every day to nourish your body with different nutrients. Make your choices as colorful as the rainbow, for each color offers a different set of nutrients that your body needs.

Chapter 2 - Tips And Tricks For Delicious Tasting Smoothies

Thick and tasty smoothies are so easy to make as long as you have a great blender. Most household blenders are actually good enough for you to use in making your smoothies.

The Blender

The blender is the main key to delicious tasting smoothies, so take heed of the following tips on how to find a really good blender (in case you do not already have one):

- **Choose a glass container.** Plastic is budget-friendly, but might discolor your smoothie and absorb odor. On the other hand, stainless steel is pretty expensive.

- **Choose the size that fits for your needs.** If you will be blending for yourself, then choose an 8-ounce blender container. If you and your significant other are sharing this smoothie journey together, then choose the 18 to 24-ounce container. If you are whipping up a batch for a family, then a 64 to 80-ounce will do.

- **Choose one with a good motor.** The average blender is powered from 300 to 600 watts, but if you really want to go all the way with this smoothie lifestyle, then get the one that is powered up by 1,300 watts. The more powerful the motor is, the more versatile your blender will be.

The Produce

It is very important to choose organic produce for your smoothies, because you certainly would not want to gulp down pesticides and other toxic chemicals.

If you find it difficult or too expensive to always opt for organic, then just stay away from the following non-organic produce because these contain the highest amount of pesticides: apples, blueberries, bell peppers, celery, grapes, collard and kale greens, nectarines, lettuce, potatoes, peaches, strawberries, and spinach.

To help you make the healthiest and safest smoothies, keep the following tips in mind:

- **Shop for in-season produce.** These locally grown crops have just been harvested, thus contain less additives for preservation. It is okay to substitute certain ingredients in the recipes with in-season produce. Your creativity and taste buds hold the limit.

- **Get your ingredients straight from the source.** Driving out to farmers who sell their produce is definitely well worth it. You will get to pick the freshest fruits and vegetables out there, still filled to the brim with all the goodness that your body needs.

- **Create a chart for in-season produce.** You will want to do this whole smoothie business all year round, so plan up your entire year on which produce is in-season. For instance, if winter is the season for cabbages and pears, then plan to use those in your smoothies for that time.

- **Fresh is best, frozen is second best.** Naturally, nothing beats fresh ingredients especially if they are in-season and locally grown. Always choose the "just ripe" variety, because under- or over-ripe ones tend to have lesser nutrients. If you cannot get a hold of fresh produce, then opt for the frozen variety. Frozen produce are usually processed during their "just ripe" stage, therefore most of its nutrients are still preserved by the time it gets into your blender.

Are you excited to start blending? In the next 8 chapters, you will find 120 smoothie recipes. Each recipe is good for one serving, so if you are blending for two, just double up the amount of each ingredient!

Also, keep in mind that you need to gulp up these smoothies as soon as they hit your glass in order for you to maximize their nutritional benefits. However, if the recipe includes lemon or lime juice, then they will last long enough in a tumbler for you to sip on the go.

Chapter 3 - Smoothie Recipes For Weight Loss

Cabbage Smoothie

- 1/8 head green cabbage
- 1/2 clove garlic, peeled
- 4 basil leaves
- 1/2 tomato
- 1/2 green bell pepper, de-stemmed

Blend all ingredients.

Hearty Veggie Smoothie

- 1 tomato
- 1 sprig cilantro
- 1/2 green onion
- 1/2 jalapeno pepper, de-stemmed
- 1/2 clove garlic
- 1 lime wedge, peeled

Blend all ingredients. Remove jalapeno pepper seeds to reduce spiciness. Serve in a soup bowl.

Keeps You Feeling Full

- 1/2 grapefruit, peeled and seeded
- 1 plum, pitted
- 1/2 banana, peeled
- 1 cup spinach
- 1/4 cup water

Blend all ingredients.

Light Limojito

- 1/2 lime, peeled
- 3 mint leaves
- 1/2 cucumber, cut into chunks

Puree all ingredients together.

Rich Recovery Smoothie

- 1/2 red potato, cut into chunks
- 1/2 cucumber, cut into chunks
- 1/2 stalk celery
- 1/2 cup spinach
- 1/2 yellow squash
- 1/2 cup broccoli florets

Blend all ingredients.

Fennel Surprise

- 1 carrot, with greens
- 1 cup spinach
- 1/8 bulb fennel with greens
- 1 lemon wedge, peeled
- 1/2 cucumber, cut into chunks
- 1/4 tsp cayenne

Blend all ingredients. Add tomato or lemon to adjust flavor if desired.

Super Beet Juice

- 1/2 beet
- 1/2 tomato
- 1 stalk celery
- 1/2 cucumber, cut into chunks

Blend all ingredients. Add 1/4 cup water to adjust consistency.

Vegetarian Vitality

- 1/2 cup spinach
- 1/2 small cucumber, cut into chunks
- 1 stalk celery
- 1 1/2 carrots, with greens
- 1/4 apple, cored and cut into chunks
- 1/4 cup apple juice or water

Blend all ingredients.

Green Extreme

- 1 stalk celery
- 1/2 cucumber, cut into chunks
- 1 cup spinach
- 1/2 apple, cored and cut into chunks
- 1/2 cup water

Blend all ingredients.

Tasty Green Beet

- 1/2 carrot, with greens
- 1/2 yellow beet
- 1 celery stalk

- 1/2 cucumber, cut into chunks
- 1/2 green bell pepper, de-stemmed

Blend all ingredients.

Lean, Mean and Green

- 1/4 cup water
- 1/2 cup cabbage
- 1 cup spinach
- 1/2 green apple, cored and cut into chunks
- 1 kiwi, peeled

Blend water and cabbage, then add spinach and apple. Pulse well. Add kiwi and puree.

Italian Slimmer

- 1/2 clove garlic
- 1/2 green bell pepper, de-stemmed
- 3 basil leaves
- 1 ripe tomato

Blend all ingredients. Add a dash of sea salt if desired.

Skinny Pepper Smoothie

- 1/4 jalapeno pepper, de-stemmed
- 1/2 green bell pepper, de-stemmed
- 1/2 cucumber, cut into chunks
- 1/2 cup arugula

- 1/4 cup water

Blend all ingredients until smooth.

Slimming Veggie Smoothie

- 1/2 potato, cut into chunks
- 1/2 green onion
- 1 tomato
- 1/2 green bell pepper, de-stemmed
- 1/8 tsp black pepper
- 1 dash of cayenne pepper

Blend all ingredients.

Salsa Smoothie

- 1 green onion
- 1/8 lb wheat grass
- 1 sprig cilantro
- 1 tomato
- 1/2 lime, peeled
- 1/4 cup water

Gradually blend all ingredients following the sequence of ingredients.

Chapter 4 - Smoothie Recipes For Radiant Skin

Goodbye Acne

- 1 potato, cut into chunks
- 3 basil leaves
- 1/2 tomato

Blend all ingredients.

Stunning Skin Smoothie

- 1/2 cup broccoli florets
- 1/2 cucumber, cut into chunks
- 1/2 kale leaf
- 1/2 bell pepper, de-stemmed
- 1/2 tomato
- 1/2 celery stalk
- 1/2 cup water

Blend all ingredients.

Berry Passionate Orange

- 1/2 orange, peeled
- 1/2 cup passion fruit
- 1/2 cup mixed berries
- 1/2 carrot, with greens

Blend all ingredients and drink up instantly.

Smooth Mediterranean

- 1/4 cup water

- 1/2 zucchini,

- 1/2 cucumber, cut into chunks

- 1/4 green bell pepper, de-stemmed

- 1 sprig dill

- 1 sprig parsley

Pulse zucchini, cucumber, and water. Add bell pepper, dill, and parsley and puree.

Pleasant Puree Smoothie

- 1/2 green apple, cored and cut into chunks

- 1 kiwi, peeled

- 1 cup romaine lettuce, chopped

- 1 sprig parsley

- 1/4 cup water

Puree all ingredients.

Barefaced Beauty

- 1/8 pineapple, peeled and cut into chunks

- 1 cup spinach

- 1/2 banana, peeled

Puree all ingredients to a desired texture.

Summery Fresh Smoothie

- 1/4 cup water

- 1/2 cup broccoli florets

- 1/2 tomato

- 1 sprig parsley
- 1/2 cucumber, cut into chunks
- 1 cup arugula

Pulse broccoli and water first, then add all other ingredients and puree.

Goodbye Wrinkles

- 1/4 cup water
- 1 plum, pitted
- 1 kiwi, peeled
- 1 cup spinach
- 3 mint leaves
- 1/2 tsp grated ginger

Pulse plum, kiwi, and water first. Add spinach, mint, and grated ginger. Puree to a desired consistency.

Youthful Italiana

- 1/2 tomato
- 1/2 clove garlic
- 1/2 green bell pepper, de-stemmed
- 2 basil leaves
- 1 kale leaf

Blend all ingredients. Add water to adjust consistency.

Berry Banana Beauty

- 1/2 banana, peeled
- 3 strawberries, capped
- 1/8 cup blueberries

- 2 kiwis, peeled

- 1/2 small cucumber, cut into chunks

- 1/8 cup water

Puree all ingredients until smooth.

Cranberry Watermelon Smoothie

- 1/2 beet, with greens

- 1/2 cup cranberries

- 1/2 cup watermelon

- 1/4 cup water

Pulse beet. Add cranberries and pulse. Add watermelon and water, then blend until smooth.

Anti-Aging Tonic

- 1/2 green apple, cored and cut into chunks

- 3 asparagus tips

- 1 cup spinach

- 1/2 cucumber, cut into chunks

- 1/4 cup water

Pulse together apple and asparagus until chunky. Add spinach, cucumber, and water. Puree to a desired consistency.

Beet Up Skin Aging

- 1/2 small sweet potato, cut into chunks

- 1/2 beet, with greens

- 1/2 carrot, with greens

- 1/2 cucumber, cut into chunks

Pulse sweet potato and beet, then blend together with carrot and cucumber. Puree to a desired consistency.

Fine Lines Begone!

- 1/4 cup blueberries
- 1/4 cup blackberries
- 1/4 cup raspberries
- 1/4 cup strawberries, capped
- 1/2 apple, cored and cut into chunks
- 1/4 cup red grapes

Blend all ingredients.

Hello Gorgeous! Smoothie

- 1/2 cup blueberries
- 1/2 cup raspberries
- 1/2 cup strawberries, capped
- 1/2 cup pomegranate seeds
- 1/4 cup plain yogurt

Blend all ingredients.

Chapter 5 - Smoothie Recipes For Detoxing The Body

Banana Bonanza

- 1 ripe banana, cut into chunks
- 1/4 cup almond milk
- 1/2 cup blueberries
- 1/2 Tbsp ground flax seed
- 1/3 cup plain yogurt

Blend all ingredients to a desired consistency.

Detox and De-stress

- 1 mango, seeded and peeled
- 1/2 orange, peeled and seeded
- 1/3 cup freshly squeezed orange juice
- 1/2 cup frozen berries of your choice

Blend all ingredients until smooth.

Nuts and Berries

- 1/6 cup cranberry juice
- 1/8 cup pomegranate juice
- 1/2 cup blueberries or blackberries
- 1/2 cup frozen acai berries
- 1/6 cup silken tofu
- 1 tbsp. chopped walnuts

Blend all ingredients until smooth.

Smooth Tropics Detox Drink

- 1/2 cup coconut milk

- 1 tbsp. whey protein powder

- 1/2 cup cantaloupe, cut into chunks

- 1/2 cup frozen peach slices

- 1/2 banana

- Optional: 1/2 tbsp. chopped Brazil nuts

Blend coconut and whey protein powder first. Add banana, cantaloupe, peach, and Brazil nuts, and blend until smooth.

Cabbage Salad Smoothie

- 1 green onion

- 1 celery stalk

- 1/2 carrot, cut into chunks

- 1/2 apple, cored and cut into chunks

- 1/2 cup fresh carrot juice

- 1/4 cup plain yogurt

- 1/2 cup chopped red or green cabbage

- 1 Tbsp chopped walnuts

- 1/2 Tbsp fresh thyme leaves

Blend all ingredients until smooth.

Vegetable Soup Smoothie

- 1/4 cucumber, cut into chunks

- 1/2 carrot

- 1/2 cup vegetable broth

- 2 tomatoes, cored and quartered
- 1/2 cup chopped kale or chard
- 1/4 cup cilantro or parsley

Blend all ingredients until smooth.

Brocco Berry

- 1/4 cup fresh carrot juice
- 1/4 cup applesauce
- 1/4 cup plain yogurt
- 1/2 cup lightly steamed broccoli
- 1/2 cup frozen blueberries
- 1/8 tsp nutmeg

Blend all ingredients until smooth.

Tomato Detox

- 1 small zucchini, peeled and cut into chunks
- 1/2 red or green bell pepper, seeds and membrane removed
- 1/2 cup fresh tomato juice
- 1 Tbsp fresh lemon juice
- 1/8 cup fresh parsley leaves
- 1 tomato, quartered
- 1/2 Tbsp freshly grated ginger

Blend all ingredients together until smooth.

Apple Detox

- 1/2 green apple, cored and cut into chunks
- 1 sprig mint

- 1 lemon wedge, peeled
- 1/2 orange, peeled
- 1/4 cucumber, quartered

Puree all ingredients to a desired consistency.

Dandelion and Kale Detox

- 1 cup dandelion greens
- 1 kale leaf
- 1/2 apple, cored and cut into chunks
- 1/2 cucumber, cut into chunks
- 2 stalks celery

Blend all ingredients until smooth.

Fennel Cleanser

- 1/2 clove garlic, peeled
- 1/8 bulb fennel, with greens
- 1 kale leaf
- 4 basil leaves
- 1/2 tomato, cut into chunks
- 1/2 cucumber, cut into chunks
- 1 lemon wedge, peeled

Blend all ingredients until smooth.

Deep Green Cleanse

- 1/2 green bell pepper, de-stemmed
- 1/2 cup broccoli florets
- 1/2 cucumber, cut into chunks

- 1/8 head cabbage

Blend all ingredients until smooth. Add more cucumber to adjust consistency and taste.

Spinach Craze

- 1 cup spinach
- 1 lemon wedge, peeled
- 1/2 sprig parsley
- 1 stalk celery

Blend all ingredients until smooth.

Super Liver Cleanse

- 1/2 beet, with greens
- 1/2 carrot, with greens
- 1/2 inch slice ginger root
- 1/2 apple, cored and cut into chunks
- 1/4 cup water
- 1/8 tsp cinnamon

Blend beet, carrot, ginger root, apple, and water together until smooth. Add cinnamon and stir.

Chili Pineapple Orange Detox

- 1/2 orange, peeled
- 1/8 pineapple, peeled
- 1 carrot, cut into chunks
- 1/4 tsp cayenne pepper

Blend all ingredients together until smooth.

Chapter 6 - Smoothie Recipes To Boost Metabolism

Celery Pineapple Boost

- 1/8 pineapple, peeled and cut into chunks
- 2 stalks celery
- 1/2 cucumber, cut into chunks

Blend all ingredients until smooth.

Ginger Snap

- 1/2 inch slice ginger root
- 1/2 carrot, with greens
- 1/2 apple, cored and cut into chunks
- 1/2 lemon, peeled

Blend all ingredients together.

Easy Sugar Treat

- 1/2 cup strawberries, capped
- 1/2 cup blueberries
- 1 carrot
- 1/2 cup wheat grass
- 1/2 beet
- 1/2 tsp cinnamon
- 1/4 cup water

Blend all ingredients together until smooth.

Ab Crunch Smoothie

- 1 sprig mint
- 1/8 inch slice ginger root
- 1/2 lime, peeled
- 1/4 bulb fennel
- 1/2 cucumber, cut into chunks
- 1/2 apple, cored and cut into chunks

Blend all ingredients together until smooth.

Melon Cranberry Metabolism

- 1/2 cup cranberries
- 1 cup watermelon
- 1/2 cup spinach

Blend all ingredients until smooth.

Green Machine

- 1 small bunch watercress
- 1 carrot
- 1/2 tomato
- 3 basil leaves
- 1/2 cup broccoli florets
- 1/2 green onion
- 1/4 cup water

Puree all ingredients together. Serve in a soup bowl.

Arugula Energy Drink

- 1/8 pineapple, peeled and cut into chunks
- 1 cup arugula

- 1/2 banana, peeled
- 1/4 cup water

Blend all ingredients together until smooth.

Extra Blast

- 1/8 pineapple, peeled and cut into chunks
- Seeds from 1/2 pomegranate
- 1/2 cup blueberries
- 1 cup spinach

Blend all ingredients until smooth.

The Wake Up Call

- 1/8 pineapple, peeled and cut into chunks
- 1/2 cup strawberries, capped
- 1/2 banana, peeled
- 1/2 cup watermelon
- 1 kiwi, peeled
- 1/4 cucumber, cut into chunks

Puree pineapple, strawberries, and banana. Add watermelon, kiwi, and cucumber and puree to a desired consistency.

Kid's Energy

- 1/2 cup cantaloupe, peeled and seeded
- 1/2 carrot, with greens
- 1 apricot, pitted
- 1/4 cup broccoli florets

Blend ingredients together until smooth.

Pink Goddess

- 1/8 pineapple, peeled and cut into chunks
- 1 plum, seeded
- 1/2 cup sour cherries, pitted
- 1/4 beet
- 1/4 cup almond milk

Blend all ingredients until smooth.

Smooth Operator

- 1/2 cup honeydew, peeled and seeded
- 1/2 cup red grapes
- 1/2 green apple, cored and cut into chunks
- 1/2 avocado, pitted and peeled

Blend all ingredients until smooth.

Monkey Wrench

- 1/2 banana, peeled
- 1/2 apple, cored and cut into chunks
- 1/2 carrot, with greens
- 1/2 cup plain or vanilla yogurt

Blend all ingredients until smooth.

Go Getter Active

- 5 fresh strawberries, capped
- 1/2 banana, peeled
- 1/4 cup broccoli florets
- 1/4 cup apple juice

- 1/4 cup blueberries
- 1/4 cup plain or vanilla yogurt

Blend all ingredients until smooth.

Beach Body Boost

- 1/8 pineapple, peeled and cut into chunks
- 1/2 avocado, pitted and peeled
- 1/2 cup mango, pitted and peeled
- 1/2 banana, peeled
- 1/4 cup pineapple juice

Blend all ingredients until smooth.

Chapter 7 - Smoothie Recipes For Increased Energy

Nutty Chocolate

- 1/2 scoop chocolate whey protein
- 1/2 banana, peeled
- 1/4 cup rolled oats
- 1 Tbsp almond butter
- 1/2 cup coconut water or water

Blend all ingredients until smooth.

Plum Energy

- 1/2 scoop vanilla whey protein
- 1/2 plum, pitted
- 1/2 banana, peeled
- 1/2 cup water
- 1/4 cup ice cubes

Blend all ingredients until smooth.

Pom Pom Cherry Smoothie

- 1/2 cup pomegranate seeds
- 1/4 cup sour cherries, pitted
- 1 kiwi, peeled
- 1/4 cup blackberries
- 1 beet
- 1/4 cup water

Blend all ingredients together until smooth.

Energy Recovery

- 1/2 cup broccoli florets
- 1/2 cup spinach
- 1/2 apple, cored and cut into chunks
- 3 kale leaves
- 1/2 banana, peeled

Blend all ingredients until smooth.

Citrus Berry Boost

- 1/8 pineapple, peeled and cut into chunks
- 1/4 cup orange juice
- 2 strawberries, capped
- 1/4 cup almond milk

Blend all ingredients until smooth.

Power Up Juice

- 1 sweet potato, cut into chunks
- 1 carrot
- 1/2 cup cantaloupe, peeled and seeded
- 1/2 cup vanilla Greek yogurt

Blend all ingredients until smooth.

Pumpkin Juice

- 1/2 sweet potato, cut into chunks
- 1/2 carrot
- 1/4 cup pumpkin

- 1/8 avocado, pitted and peeled

- 1/4 cup almond or soy milk

- Optional: a dash of cinnamon

Blend carrots and sweet potato first, then add pumpkin, avocado, and almond or soy milk. Blend until smooth. Add a dash of cinnamon and stir.

Great Guava Smoothie

- 1/2 guava, peeled

- 1/8 cantaloupe, peeled and seeded

- 1/2 carrot, with greens

- 1/4 cup coconut milk

Blend all ingredients until smooth.

Summer Radiance

- 1 plum, pitted

- 1 cup watermelon

- 1/2 small cucumber, cut into chunks

Blend all ingredients until smooth.

Berry Guava Grape Smoothie

- 1/2 guava, peeled

- 1/2 cup watermelon

- 1/2 cup red grapes

- 1/2 cup raspberries

Blend all ingredients until smooth.

Carrot Spinach Smoothie

- 1/4 sweet potato, cut into chunks

- 1 cup spinach
- 1 carrot
- 1 cup apple juice

Blend all ingredients until smooth.

Citrus Spin

- 1 orange, peeled
- 1/2 lemon, peeled
- 1 grapefruit, peeled

Blend all ingredients until smooth.

Red Lemonade

- 2 lemons, peeled
- 1/4 jalapeno pepper, de-stemmed
- 1/2 cucumber, cut into chunks
- 1 cup water

Blend all ingredients until smooth.

Low Sugar, High Energy

- 1/4 sweet potato, cut into chunks
- 1/4 cup wheat grass
- 1 lemon wedge, peeled
- 1/4 cup cranberries
- 1/4 inch slice ginger root
- 1/4 cup water

Blend all ingredients until smooth.

Burn Baby, Burn

- 1/2 celery stalk

- 1/2 tomato

- 1/2 lemon, peeled

- 1 carrot

- 1/4 jalapeno pepper, de-stemmed

Blend all ingredients together until smooth. For an extra zing, make it 1/2 jalapeno pepper.

Chapter 8 - Smoothie Recipes To Strengthen Your Immune System

Immunity Shield

- 1/4 cup coconut water
- 1/4 tsp probiotic powder
- 1 Tbsp acai powder
- Optional: 1 tsp maqui powder
- 1/4 cup blueberries
- 1/4 cup blackberries
- 1/4 cup raspberries
- 1/4 cup strawberries
- 1/4 cup red seedless grapes
- 1/2 ripe pear, cored and diced
- 1/4 tsp minced ginger root
- 1/8 tsp ground cinnamon
- 1/4 tsp finely grated orange zest
- 1/2 cup ice cubes
- 1/2 pitted date, chopped and soaked in water overnight

Puree all ingredients until creamy and smooth.

Kale Ice Cream

- 1/4 cup water
- 1/4 tsp probiotic powder
- 1/4 cup raw unsalted cashews, soaked in water overnight

- 1/2 cup torn up kale leaves

- 1 ripe banana, peeled

- 1/8 cup chopped pitted dates, soaked overnight

Place ingredients into the blender following the sequence given. Puree until creamy and smooth.

Lemon Raspberry Cheesecake

- 1/2 cup coconut water or water

- 1/4 tsp probiotic powder

- 1/3 cup raw unsalted cashews, soaked overnight

- 1/2 cup raspberries

- 1/4 banana, peeled

- 1 1/2 Tbsp freshly squeezed lemon juice

- 1/2 Tbsp pure maple syrup

- 1/2 tsp alcohol-free vanilla extract

- A dash of finely grated lemon zest

- A dash of natural salt

- 1/2 cup ice cubes

Blend all ingredients until smooth.

Fruit Curry

- 1 cup water

- 1/4 cup coconut milk

- 1/2 cup diced mango

- 1/2 cup diced pineapple

- 1/2 cup diced peaches

- 1/4 tsp finely grated lime zest

- 1 cup ice cubes

- 1/4 tsp yellow curry powder

- A dash of red pepper flakes

- A dash of natural salt

- 1/2 Tbsp pure maple syrup

Blend all ingredients together until smooth and creamy.

Creamy Orange Smoothie

- 3/4 cup freshly squeezed orange juice

- 1/4 tsp probiotic powder

- 1/2 orange, peeled and seeded

- 1/2 cup roughly chopped strawberries

- 1/4 cup diced red bell pepper

- 1/4 cup roughly chopped baked or steamed orange sweet potato, peeled

- 1/4 cup frozen raw cauliflower florets

- 1/8 cup firm silken tofu

- 1/8 cup blanched, slivered raw almonds, soaked in water overnight

- 1 tsp finely grated orange zest

- 1/2 tsp alcohol-free vanilla extract

- A dash of ground turmeric

- 1/2 Tbsp pure maple syrup

- 1 cup ice cubes

- 1/2 tsp ground flax seeds
- Optional: 1/2 dried apricot, finely chopped
- Optional: 1/2 Tbsp dried goji berries

Blend all ingredients together until smooth and creamy.

Papaya Blend

- 1/2 cup unsweetened almond milk
- 1 cup roughly chopped papaya
- 1/4 cup roughly chopped mango
- 1 tsp freshly squeezed lemon juice
- 1 tsp minced ginger root
- 1/2 tsp flax seed oil
- A dash of ground cinnamon
- A dash of finely grated lemon zest
- 1/8 tsp alcohol-free vanilla extract
- 3 drops alcohol-free liquid stevia
- 1/2 cup ice cubes

Blend all ingredients together until smooth and creamy. Add more ginger, cinnamon or lemon zest to adjust the flavor.

Mint Green Immunity Booster

- 1/2 cup unsweetened almond milk
- 1/2 cup coconut water
- 1/2 Tbsp vanilla protein powder
- 1/4 tsp probiotic powder
- 1/2 tsp wheat grass powder

- 1/4 tsp spirulina powder
- 1/4 tsp chlorella powder
- 1 cup firmly packed baby spinach
- 1 cup frozen sliced banana
- 1/3 cup raw unsalted cashews, soaked in water overnight
- 1/8 cup firmly packed mint leaves
- 1/2 tsp alcohol-free vanilla extract
- Optional: 1/8 tsp peppermint extract
- 1/2 Tbsp coconut nectar
- 1/2 cup ice cubes

Blend all ingredients until smooth.

Asparagus Tonic
- 1 tsp olive oil
- 1/4 tsp minced garlic
- 1/4 cup chopped leeks, white parts only
- A dash of natural salt
- 1/8 cup diced celery
- 1/4 cup diced green zucchini
- 1/4 cup diced long yellow squash
- 1/4 cup chopped cauliflower florets
- 1 cup vegetable broth
- 1 cup chopped asparagus
- 1 tsp chopped flat leaf parsley

- 1 Tbsp blanched slivered raw almonds, soaked in water overnight

- 1/4 tsp freshly squeezed lemon juice

Saute olive oil, garlic, and leeks over medium heat. Season with salt. Add celery, zucchini, squash, and cauliflower. Saute until soft. Add vegetable broth and bring to a boil. Reduce heat, let simmer. Add asparagus and parsley. Simmer for 5 minutes until tender.

Set aside to cool. Add almonds. Pour soup into blender and puree until smooth and creamy. Warm over medium heat, if preferred. Serve in a soup bowl.

Probiotic Kefir

- 1/2 cup unsweetened almond milk

- 1/2 cup coconut milk kefir

- 3/4 cup strawberries, capped

- 1/2 Tbsp raw almond butter

- 1/2 tsp shelled hemp seeds

- 1/2 tsp black or white chia seeds

- 1/2 tsp ground flax seeds

- 1/2 tsp alcohol-free vanilla extract

- 1/8 tsp probiotic powder

- 1/8 tsp finely grated lemon zest

- 1/1 tsp ground cinnamon

- A dash of natural salt

- 10 drops alcohol-free liquid stevia

- Optional: 1/2 cup ice cubes

Blend all ingredients until creamy and smooth.

Beat the Flu Smoothie

- 3/4 cup water

- 1 carrot, peeled and chopped

- 1/4 large or 1/2 small green apple, cored and cut into chunks

- 1/2 Tbsp freshly squeezed lemon juice

- 1 tsp minced ginger

- 1/16 tsp ground cinnamon

- A dash of cayenne pepper

- 3 drops alcohol-free liquid stevia

Blend all ingredients until smooth. Chill first before serving, if preferred.

Vegan Rose Water Lassi

- 1/2 cup coconut milk yogurt or kefir

- 1/4 cup coconut milk

- 1 sliced banana

- 1 cup ice cubes

- 1/4 tsp ground cardamom

- 1/2 tsp pure distilled rose water

- 1/2 tsp freshly squeezed lemon juice

- 1/2 pitted date, soaked in water overnight

Blend all ingredients together until smooth and creamy.

Strawberry Basil Smoothie

- 1 cup water

- 1/4 cup freshly squeezed lemon juice

- 1 1/2 cups chopped strawberries

- 1/6 cup agave nectar
- 1/8 cup firmly packed basil.

Blend all ingredients together until smooth and creamy.

Mint and Grape Smoothie

- 1 cup water
- 1/4 cup freshly squeezed lemon juice
- 2 cups green seedless grapes
- 7 mint leaves
- 1/2 Tbsp agave nectar

Blend all ingredients together until smooth and creamy. Add more lemon juice to adjust the flavor.

Ginger Pineapple Smoothie

- 1 cup water
- 1/4 cup freshly squeezed lemon juice
- 1 1/2 cups diced ripe pineapple
- 1/2 Tbsp minced ginger root
- 1 Tbsp agave nectar

Blend all ingredients together until smooth and creamy.

Chia Isotonic Drink

- 1 cup coconut water
- 1/2 tsp finely grated lime zest
- 1/8 cup freshly squeezed orange juice
- 1 Tbsp freshly squeezed lemon juice
- 1 Tbsp freshly squeezed lime juice

- 1 Tbsp black or white chia seeds

- 2 Alcohol-free liquid stevia.

Blend coconut water, zest, and juices. Add chia seeds and blend on low until well-distributed. Sweeten with liquid stevia and blend to combine.

Chapter 9 - Green Smoothie Recipes For Alkaline Weight Loss

Potato and Pineapple

- 1/2 red potato, chopped
- 1/8 pineapple, peeled and chopped
- 1/8 inch ginger root
- 1 kiwi, peeled

Pulse ginger and potato, then add kiwi and pineapple. Blend until smooth. Add 1/8 cup organic apple juice or water to adjust consistency.

Cranberry Lemon

- 1/2 cup cranberries
- 1 lemon, peeled
- 1 1/2 cups water

Blend all ingredients.

Orange and Carrot

- 1/2 yellow beet
- 1/2 carrot, with greens
- 1/2 orange, peeled
- 1/4 cup coconut water

Pulse carrot and beet first, then add orange and coconut water. Blend until smooth.

Minty Lemony Greens

- 1/2 cucumber, cut into chunks
- 1/4 bunch fresh parsley

- 1/4 lemon, peeled
- 1/2 cup alfalfa sprouts
- 2 sprigs fresh mint

Blend all ingredients.

Fabulous Red

- 1/2 beet
- 1/2 cup pomegranate seeds or cranberries
- 1/2 cup watermelon
- 1/4 lime, peeled

Pulse beet. Blend all ingredients together.

Alka-Lime

- 1 kale leaf
- 1/2 cup spinach
- 1/2 lime, peeled
- 1/2 green bell pepper, de-stemmed
- 1/2 cucumber, cut into chunks
- 1/2 carrot, with greens

Pulse lime, spinach, and kale first. Add other ingredients and blend until smooth. Add 1/4 cup water to adjust consistency.

Crisp Greens and Carrot

- 1/2 watercress
- 1/2 cup spinach
- 1/2 cup broccoli florets
- 1/2 carrot, with greens

- 1/2 cup water

Pulse watercress, spinach, and broccoli. Add other ingredients and blend until smooth.

Alkaline Ale

- 1/4 sweet potato cut into cubes
- 1/4 cup raspberries
- 1/4 cup orange, peeled
- 2 strawberries, capped
- 1/4 cucumber, cut into chunks
- Optional: 2 sprigs mint

Blend all ingredients.

Power Shake

- 1/2 clove garlic
- 1/8 head cabbage
- 1/2 kale leaf
- 1/2 beet
- 1/2 carrot
- 1/2 stalk celery
- 1/2 cup water

Blend all ingredients.

Pumpkin Spice

- 1/4 apple, cored and cut into chunks
- 1/2 cup pumpkin
- 1/2 small cucumber, cut into chunks

- 1/2 carrot
- 1/4 tsp ground cloves
- 1/4 tsp ground cinnamon

Blend all ingredients.

Pale Green Shake

- 1/2 carrot, with greens
- 1/2 apple, cored and cut into chunks
- 1/2 cucumber, cut into chunks
- 1 kale leaf

Blend all ingredients.

Peppery arugula

- 1/2 cup arugula
- 1/4 whole watercress
- 1/2 stalk celery
- 1/4 lb lemon grass
- 1/2 green bell pepper, de-stemmed
- 1/4 tsp prepared horseradish

Blend all ingredients.

Sweet Greens

- 1/2 cup broccoli florets
- 1/2 carrot, with greens
- 3 Brussels sprouts
- 1 cup spinach
- 1/2 cup water

Pulse broccoli florets, carrot, Brussels sprouts, and water. Add water and blend until smooth.

Potato Melon Delight

- 1/2 small sweet potato, chopped
- 1/2 small white potato, chopped
- 1/8 cantaloupe, peeled and seeded
- 1/8 cucumber, cut into cubes

Pulse potatoes first, then blend all ingredients.

Green Reset

- 1/2 cup broccoli florets
- 1 stalk celery
- 1 cup spinach
- 1/2 clove garlic, peeled
- 1/8 head cabbage
- 1/2 cup water

Blend all ingredients.

Chapter 10 - Healing Foods; Smoothie Recipes To Fight Cancers & Diseases

Minty Berry Cherry

- 1/2 cup cherries, pitted
- 2 sprigs mint
- 1/4 cucumber, chopped
- 1/2 cup raspberries
- 1/2 apple, cored and cut into chunks

Blend ingredients together. Add 1/4 cup coconut water to adjust consistency.

Health Booster

- 1/4 sweet potato, cubed
- 1 cup spinach
- 1/2 clove garlic
- 1/2 carrot, with greens
- 1/4 small cucumber, cut into chunks
- 1/4 cup water

Pulse sweet potato, spinach, garlic, then blend all ingredients. Add more cucumber for a lighter flavor.

Tropical Mint

- 1/4 mango, pitted and peeled
- 2 sprigs mint
- 1/2 cup pomegranate
- 1/8 papaya, seeded and peeled

- 1/4 cup almond milk

Blend ingredients together.

Apple Cherry

- 1/2 apple, cored and cut into chunks
- 1/2 cup sour cherries, pitted
- 1 sprig mint
- 1 oz seltzer water

Blend apple, cherries, and mint. Add seltzer water and pulse to blend.

Smoothie Gazpacho

- 1/4 cup water
- 1 clove garlic, peeled
- 1/2 cucumber, cut into chunks
- 1/2 avocado, pitted and peeled
- 1/2 green bell pepper, de-stemmed
- Optional: 1 small jalapeno pepper, de-stemmed
- 1 small zucchini, cut into chunks
- 1 scallion
- 1/2 tsp lime juice

Blend garlic, cucumber, avocado, and water. Add other ingredients and blend until smooth. Serve in a soup bowl.

Tropical Buffet

- 1/8 pineapple, peeled and cubed
- 1/8 cantaloupe, peeled and seeded
- 1/2 cup spinach

- 1/2 orange, peeled
- 1/2 cup pomegranate seeds

Blend all ingredients.

Greens Lover

- 3 kale leaves
- 1/2 cup spinach
- 1/2 cup collard greens
- 1/2 green bell pepper, de-stemmed
- 1/2 clove garlic
- 1/2 cup water

Blend ingredients. Season with black pepper and sea salt if desired.

Artichoke Broccoli

- 1/2 cup broccoli florets
- 1/2 artichoke heart
- 1/2 carrot, with greens
- 1/2 clove garlic
- 1/2 small cucumber, cut into chunks

Blend ingredients together. Add 1/2 cup water to adjust consistency.

Green Booster

- 1 stalk celery
- 1/2 green bell pepper, de-stemmed
- 2 asparagus tips, broken up
- 1/2 lemon, peeled

- Optional: 1/2 jalapeno pepper, de-stemmed

For less spiciness, remove jalapeno pepper seeds. Blend all ingredients.

Sleeper Smoothie

- 1/4 cup cherries, frozen
- 1/2 pear, cored and cut into chunks
- 1/2 apple, cored and cut into chunks
- 1/4 zucchini
- 1/4 inch ginger root
- 1/2 carrot
- 1/2 cup spinach
- 1/4 cup water

Blend all ingredients.

Cucumber Carrot

- 1/2 cucumber, cut into chunks
- 1/2 carrot, with greens
- 1/2 apple, cored and cut into chunks
- 1/2 lemon, peeled

Blend all ingredients.

Autumn Harvest

- 1/2 sweet potato, cut into chunks
- 1/2 cup pumpkin
- 1/2 apple, cored and cut into chunks
- 1/2 tsp cinnamon

- 1/4 inch ginger root

- 1/2 carrot

- 1/4 cup water

Blend all ingredients.

Ginger Fizz

- 1 kiwi, peeled

- 1/2 stalk celery

- 1/4 inch ginger root

- 1/2 cucumber, cut into chunks

- 1/2 apple, cored and cut into chunks

- 1/2 cup sour cherries, pitted

- 1/4 cup sparkling water

Blend all ingredients.

Blueberry Explosion

- 1/2 cup blueberries

- 1/2 cup blackberries

- 1/2 cucumber, cut into chunks

Blend all ingredients. Add 1/4 cup almond milk to adjust consistency.

Very Berry and Cherry

- 1/2 cup dark cherries, pitted

- 1/2 cup blueberries

- 1/2 cup raspberries

- 1/4 lemon, peeled

- 1/2 cucumber, cut into chunks

Blend all ingredients.

Conclusion

Thank you again for purchasing this book on Smoothie Recipes!

I am extremely excited to pass this information along to you, and I am so happy that you now have read and can hopefully implement these strategies going forward.

I hope this book was able to help you understand the process of making healthy smoothies and how to start whipping up your own at home.

The next step is to get started using this information and to hopefully live a healthy and happy life!

Please don't be someone who just reads this information and doesn't apply it, the strategies in this book will only benefit you if you use them!

If you know of anyone else that could benefit from the information presented here please inform them of this book.

Finally, if you enjoyed this book and feel it has added value to your life in any way, please take the time to share your thoughts and post a review on Amazon. It'd be greatly appreciated!

Thank you and good luck!

Preview Of:

Ultimate Paleo Diet For Beginners!

Paleo

Instant Paleo Weight Loss Tips And Recipes To Get In Shape, Lose Weight, Build Muscle, And Transform Your Body Fast!

Introduction

I want to thank you and congratulate you for purchasing the book, *Paleo: Ultimate Paleo Diet For Beginners! Instant Paleo Weight Loss Tips And Recipes To Get In Shape, Lose Weight, Build Muscle, And Transform Your Body Fast!*

This book contains proven steps and strategies on how to lose weight effectively and keep your body strong and healthy. It is true that what we eat affects our overall health. Having said that, it is important that we know what we eat and consume only foods that are good for our body.

The Paleo diet allows you to eat all the foods that you want, without sacrificing taste and nutrition. Many people wonder how a caveman diet can be done during these modern times. It may not be easy at first, but this book will help you decide which foods are good for you and which are not.

In this book, you will:

- Learn how to choose foods that are Paleo-accepted.

- Know the benefits of Paleo diet and how it affects your health.

- Learn how to use Paleo effectively to build muscles and lose weight fast and effectively.

Although many diets are out there, the Paleo Diet has been proven effective by many and it has stood the tests of time. Even skeptics have seen the light and realized how beneficial the Paleo Diet is.

Thanks again for purchasing this book, I hope you enjoy it!

Chapter 1: Paleo Basics – What Does It Mean To Eat Paleo?

The Paleo Diet, short for Paleolithic Age Diet, aims to mimic the diet that our ancestors had long before agriculture came to the scene. During the Paleolithic era, our ancestors hunt their food, meaning they only eat free-range animals and any available fruits and vegetables in the wild. In our modern times, the Paleo diet means consuming grass-fed animals and organic fruits and vegetables. It's hard to replicate the caveman diet precisely; but the core idea is to eat unprocessed whole foods that contain all the proteins, nutrients and even the carbohydrates that our body needs.

Paleo diet means dumping the processed, refined, genetically-modified fruits, vegetables and meat and replacing them with farm-raised animals, fruits and vegetables. Note that most modern diseases such as autoimmune diseases, cancer and Type II Diabetes started to surface after industrialized foods or processed foods took upon the shelves of supermarkets and groceries.

Contrary to what many people know, finding the proper ingredients suitable for Paleo diet is not that hard. In fact, when you choose to go Paleo, you are actually helping small farmers make a better living. Paleo ingredients are often found in the farmer's markets. In general, small farmers grow their own fruits and vegetables in their small lands and usually use the traditional way of farming. Farm animals are also grown traditionally and are free from chemicals that are usually injected to commercial animals for them to be processed into foods at an earlier time.

Some farmers may use pesticides in their crops. This is something you should watch out for. Therefore, the best way to ensure that you are getting the best is to use organic foods. They are much more expensive, but the health and nutrition they provide is none compared to the money you spend. In case you can't get hold of organic foods, just make sure to stay away from any processed foods, sugar, legumes and grains that contain gluten.

Following the Paleo diet plan is not that hard. You don't even need to count your calories, nor do you need to give up your favorite foods. You just need to substitute unhealthy foods with whole unprocessed ones. The good news is that Paleo foods are tasty and packed with all the nutrients that you need.

Benefits of the Paleo diet

The following are some of the benefits that you will gain from sticking to a Paleo diet:

- Sustained weight loss

- Increased energy

- Increased muscle growth and fitness

- Reduced risk of diabetes, cancer and heart diseases

- Better nutrient absorption

- Higher immunity

- Improved glucose tolerance

- Healthy cells and brain

- Better digestion and gut health

- Reduced inflammation and allergies

- Increased sensitivity to insulin

- Reduced bloating

Thanks for Previewing My Exciting Book Entitled:

"Paleo: Instant Paleo Weight Loss Tips And Recipes To Get In Shape, Lose Weight, Build Muscle, And Transform Your Body Fast!"

To purchase this book, simply go to the Amazon Kindle store and simply search:

"PALEO"

Then just scroll down until you see my book. You will know it is mine because you will see my name "Sarah Brooks" underneath the title.

Alternatively, you can visit my author page on Amazon to see this book and other work I have done. Thanks so much, and please don't forget your free bonuses

DON'T LEAVE YET! - CHECK OUT YOUR FREE BONUSES BELOW!

Free Bonus Offer: Get Free Access To The www.LiveFitVIP.com VIP Newsletter!

Once you enter your email address you will immediately get free access to this awesome newsletter!

But wait, right now if you join now for free you will also get free access to the "The 7 Keys To Body Transformation" free EBook!

To claim both your FREE VIP NEWSLETTER MEMBERSHIP and your FREE BONUS Ebook on THE 7 KEYS TO BODY TRANSFORMATION!

Just Go To:

www.liveFitVIP.com